Morgane Lee Rice

BEYOND THE BASICS

'Exploring Sexuality and Empowering Girls to make Informed Choices'

CHAPTER 3

Condoms:
Hormonal Contraception
Long-Acting Reversible Contraception (LARCs)
Emergency contraception
STI Prevention
Dual Protection
Consultation with Healthcare Professionals
3.4 PREVENTING SEXUALLY TRANSMITTED INFECTIONS (STIS)
SEXUALLY TRANSMITTED DISEASES (STIS)
a) Human Immunodeficiency Virus (HIV):
b) Chlamydia
c) Gonorrhea:
d) Syphilis:
e) Genital Herpes:
f) Human Papillomavirus (HPV):
g) Hepatitis B and C:
PREVENTION STRATEGIES:
a) Abstinence:
b) Condom Use:
c) Vaccination:
c) STI Testing:
e) discussion and Trust:
f) Reducing the Number of Sexual Partners
g) Safe Injection Practices
h) Prenatal Care:
The Value of Early Diagnosis and Treatment
3.5 MAKING INFORMED SEXUAL ACTIVITY AND READINESS DECISIONS
Self-Reflection:
Emotional Preparedness:
Communication and Consent:
Education and Awareness:
Recognize and resist peer pressure and societal expectations around sexual activity
Consider the characteristics of your relationship
Personal Boundaries:
Seeking Advice:

CONCLUSION

Introduction

"Beyond the Basics: Exploring Sexuality and Empowering Girls to Make Informed Choices." This book is here to be your companion, providing you with the knowledge and guidance you need to make the best decisions about sex education tailored specifically for girls. We believe that every girl deserves to be informed, empowered to make informed choices, and supported in her journey of sexual wellness. We know that understanding and embracing our sexuality can be a complex and sometimes overwhelming experience. It's normal to have questions and concerns about sex, relationships, and our bodies, and this book aims to create a safe and inclusive space where you can explore these topics without judgment. In the pages that follow, we'll cover a wide range of essential subjects. We'll start by unraveling the mysteries of puberty and the physical changes that come with it.

Then, we'll dive into building healthy relationships and effective communication skills, so you can set boundaries and recognize signs of unhealthy dynamics. We'll also delve into the realms of sexuality, pleasure, and self-discovery, guiding you on understanding your desires, embracing self-pleasure, and navigating consent and safe sexual practices. We'll also address the importance of contraception and the prevention of sexually transmitted infections, so you can prioritize your sexual health.

Throughout this book, we want you to approach these topics with an open mind and a sense of curiosity. We'll present information in a non-judgmental manner, respecting individual choices and perspectives. Everyone's experiences and beliefs may differ, and it's important to find what feels right for you. Knowledge is power, and by arming yourself with accurate information and the tools to make informed choices, you can confidently navigate the path of sexual empowerment. We hope that this book will serve as a valuable resource, offering guidance, support, and encouragement as you embark on this journey of self-discovery.

So, let's embark on this empowering expedition together, embracing our bodies, our desires, and our right to make informed choices. Let's unlock the potential within us and redefine the narrative around sex education for girls. Together, we can navigate the complexities, celebrate our individuality, and emerge as empowered individuals ready to embrace a fulfilling and healthy sexual journey.

Chapter 1

Understanding your Body and Sexual Development

1.1 What is Puberty?

Puberty is a natural and normal process that marks the start of sexual maturation and the transition from childhood to adolescence. It is a complex combination of physical, hormonal, and psychological changes that occur in both boys and girls as their bodies prepare for adulthood.

Puberty usually begins between the ages of 8 and 13 in girls, although the timing can vary for each individual.

The body undergoes a major transformation during puberty, as it matures sexually. This is guided by hormones released by the hypothalamus in the brain, which stimulate the ovaries in girls to produce the female sex hormones, estrogen and progesterone. These hormones cause a series of changes throughout the body, which can take several years to complete. The start of puberty is often marked by physical changes and the beginning of the menstrual cycle, known as menarche. In addition to physical changes, puberty also brings about emotional, social, and cognitive transformations. Adolescents experience heightened emotions, increased self-awareness, and a growing desire for independence. It is a time of self-discovery, identity formation, and exploring new experiences and relationships. It is important to remember that puberty is a highly individualized process.

The timing, duration, and pace of puberty can vary significantly from person to person. Some girls may begin puberty earlier or later than their peers, and the rate of development can also differ. It is essential to approach puberty with patience and understanding, recognizing that each person's journey is unique. Understanding what puberty is and the changes it brings is essential for girls as they go through this transformative period. By learning about the physical, hormonal, and emotional changes that occur during puberty, girls can develop a sense of empowerment and self-acceptance, enabling them to embrace this natural progression with confidence and resilience. The timeline of puberty refers to the sequence of events and the general age range at which different physical and hormonal changes typically occur in girls.

1.2 The timeline of Puberty

It's important to remember that the timeline can vary from person to person, and individual differences are entirely normal. However, understanding the general patterns can provide a helpful framework for girls to anticipate and navigate the changes they may experience during puberty.

Early puberty: This is also known as prepubertal or early-stage puberty, which generally begins between the ages of 8 and 11. During this phase, the body starts preparing for the forthcoming physical changes. Some of the initial signs of early puberty in girls may include breast buds, the growth of fine, straight hair in the pubic area, increased sweat production, and changes in sweat composition, leading to body odor.

Mid-puberty: This usually occurs between the ages of 11 and 14. This is when significant physical changes take place as the body continues its development. Key milestones during mid-puberty include a rapid increase in height, the onset of the menstrual cycle, fuller breast development, and an accumulation of body fat, particularly around the hips, buttocks, and thighs.

Late Puberty: Also known as post-puberty or late-stage puberty, usually happens between the ages of 14 and 16. By this point, most of the physical changes associated with puberty have already taken place. Some of the developments during late puberty include the completion of breast development, pubic hair growth, and the maturation of reproductive organs. It's important to remember that the timeline provided is just a general guideline, and individual variations are normal.

Factors such as genetics, ethnicity, overall health, and environmental factors can all influence the age at which puberty begins and progresses. That's why it's so important for girls to focus on their unique journey through puberty and not compare themselves to others. Understanding the timeline of puberty can help girls anticipate and accept the changes they may experience, while also providing them with the reassurance that the physical transformations they go through are a normal part of their development into adulthood.

1.3 Physical changes during Puberty

Puberty is a period of significant physical changes as the body matures sexually. These changes occur gradually over time and are primarily driven by the hormone's estrogen and progesterone. Girls may experience a variety of physical changes during this time, including breast development, body hair growth, growth spurts, skin changes, body shape, and fat distribution, increased sweat and odor, and voice changes. Each individual's journey through puberty is unique, and there is a wide range of normal variations. It is important to remember that these changes are natural and normal, and girls should embrace their evolving bodies with confidence and self-acceptance.

Breast development: This development is one of the earliest signs of puberty in girls, with the breasts beginning to grow as glandular tissue and fat accumulate beneath the nipples. Over time, the breasts become fuller and more rounded, and the areolas may also enlarge and darken.

Body hair: During puberty, girls will notice the growth of hair in various parts of their bodies, such as the pubic area, underarms, legs, and sometimes arms and upper lip. As girls go through puberty, they experience a rapid growth spurt, typically occurring around the age of 12.

Growth Spurts: During this period, girls may experience a significant increase in height and changes in body proportions.

Skin changes: Skin changes are also common during puberty, with increased oil production leading to oily skin and potential acne breakouts. Establishing a skincare routine can help manage skin changes.

Body Shape and fat distribution: Puberty also brings about changes in body shape due to the redistribution of fat, with girls typically experiencing an increase in body fat, particularly in the hips, buttocks, and thighs.

Sweat and Odor: Sweat glands become more active during puberty, leading to increased perspiration and body odor. Girls may need to use deodorant or antiperspirant to manage body odor and maintain personal hygiene.

Voice changes: These are more prominent in boys during puberty, but girls may also experience some slight changes in their voice. The vocal cords thicken and lengthen, causing a subtle deepening of the voice. Understanding these changes can help girls feel more confident and self-accepting of their bodies as they go through this natural and normal process of growth and development.

1.4 The Role of Hormones

Hormones are essential for the physical and physiological changes that occur during puberty. In girls, two primary hormones, estrogen, and progesterone, are responsible for the development and maturation of reproductive organs and secondary sexual characteristics.

Let's take a closer look at the role of these hormones during puberty:

Estrogen: Estrogen is the main female sex hormone produced mainly in the ovaries. Its levels increase significantly during puberty and are essential for various aspects of development.

Some of the key functions of estrogen include:

- Breast development: Estrogen stimulates the growth of breast tissue, leading to the formation of breast buds and subsequent breast development. It also promotes the accumulation of fat in the breasts and increases blood flow to the area.

- Growth and skeletal development: Estrogen contributes to the growth plates in bones, helping promote bone growth and maturation. It also plays a role in determining the timing of the growth spurt during puberty.
- Fat distribution: Estrogen influences the redistribution of body fat, causing an increase in subcutaneous fat deposition in the hips, buttocks, and thighs. This contributes to the development of a more curvaceous body shape.
- Development of reproductive organs: Estrogen stimulates the growth and maturation of the uterus, fallopian tubes, and vagina, preparing them for potential pregnancy. It also promotes the thickening and vascularization of the uterine lining (endometrium) in preparation for menstruation.
- Progesterone: Progesterone is another hormone produced in the ovaries, particularly in the second half of the menstrual cycle. Its primary role is to support pregnancy and regulate the menstrual cycle. During puberty, progesterone levels remain relatively low compared to estrogen.

Some of the key functions of progesterone include:

- Regulation of the menstrual cycle: Progesterone works in conjunction with estrogen to regulate the menstrual cycle. It helps prepare the uterus for potential pregnancy by maintaining the thickened uterine lining (endometrium) after ovulation.
- Modulation of mood and emotions: Progesterone affects neurotransmitters in the brain, which can influence mood and emotions. It can have calming and stabilizing effects, although the exact mechanisms are complex and not fully understood.

It's important to note that other hormones, such as follicle-stimulating hormone (FSH) and luteinizing hormone (LH) released by the pituitary gland, also play significant roles in initiating and regulating the hormonal changes of puberty. FSH stimulates the growth of ovarian follicles and the production of estrogen, while LH triggers ovulation and the subsequent release of progesterone.

These hormones work together in a carefully orchestrated feedback system, with the hypothalamus, pituitary gland, and ovaries communicating to maintain hormonal balance and coordinate the physiological changes of puberty. Understanding the role of hormones during puberty helps girls understand the intricate mechanisms driving their physical development. It also emphasizes the importance of hormonal balance for overall health and well-being.

1.5 Emotional and Psychological Alterations

Puberty is more than simply physical changes; it also brings about a variety of emotional and psychological changes. Adolescent hormone surges, paired with social and cognitive developments, can have a substantial impact on a girl's emotional well-being and self-perception.

Here are some of the most frequent emotional and psychological changes that occur during puberty:

Mood Swings: Hormone fluctuations throughout puberty can contribute to mood swings. Girls' emotions can shift quickly and intensely, from happiness and enthusiasm to sadness, impatience, or wrath. These mood swings are a natural aspect of puberty's emotional roller coaster.

Increased Self-Awareness: As females enter puberty, they often become more self-conscious and aware of their bodies, appearance, and social interactions. They may compare themselves to others and have increased self-awareness, which can lead to emotions of self-doubt or uneasiness. During this time, it is critical to promote self-acceptance and a positive body image.

Identity Formation: Adolescence is a vital time for identity development. Girls may investigate several parts of their identity, such as their values, interests, beliefs, and connections. They may become more self-aware and question their place in the world. Experimentation, trying out new roles, and creating personal ideals can all be part of the self-discovery process.

Peer Relationships: Changes in peer dynamics are common during puberty. Girls may want to make new friends or negotiate to change connections with old ones. Peer pressure increases, and social approval and belonging may become more important. Girls may experience the pleasures of developing close friendships as well as the difficulties of navigating disagreements and social pressures.

Cognitive Development and Changes in Thinking Patterns: Puberty is also connected with cognitive development and changes in thinking patterns. Girls' ability to think abstractly, evaluate many views, and participate in critical thinking may improve. Individuals' cognitive growth may not be uniform, and they may progress at varying speeds.

Sexual and Romantic Interest: As girls reach puberty, they may develop sexual and romantic feelings. They may become interested in relationships, attracted to others, or curious about sexuality. Exploring and comprehending new feelings is a natural component of adolescent growth.

It is crucial to remember that the emotional and psychological changes that occur during puberty can differ greatly among individuals. Some females may find this period easy, while others may find it difficult. Open and supportive contact with trustworthy adults, such as parents, caregivers, or mentors, can provide the assistance and comfort that girls require to effectively manage these transitions.

Promoting good self-esteem, encouraging self-care routines, and cultivating healthy coping skills are critical for supporting girls' emotional well-being during puberty. We can help girls build resilience, self-acceptance, and the skills needed to traverse this transformative time of their lives by fostering a supportive environment that respects the emotional and psychological changes that are occurring.

Chapter 2

Building healthy relationships and communication

2.1 Boundaries and Consent Are Important

Boundaries and permission are important concepts that allow people to keep control over their bodies, emotions, and personal interactions. Understanding and maintaining boundaries, as well as obtaining consent, are essential for developing healthy relationships, supporting autonomy, and avoiding harm. Here's more on the significance of boundaries and consent:

Boundaries and Consent: Boundaries and consent acknowledge and respect people's autonomy and personal agency. They acknowledge that everyone has the freedom to make decisions regarding their bodies, emotions, and personal interactions. Individuals can assert their preferences, desires, and limits without feeling coerced or violated when boundaries are respected and consent is obtained.

Harm and Abuse Prevention: Boundaries and consent serve as protective measures against harm as well as exploitation. They create a framework for healthy partnerships by requiring voluntary and mutually respectful exchanges. Clear boundaries assist individuals in establishing limits and communicating their level of comfort, lowering the danger of physical, mental, or sexual harm. Consent ensures that all parties are willing participants and that no one is subjected to undesired or nonconsensual activities.

Boundaries and consent promote open and honest communication within relationships, which improves communication and trust. Individuals can convey their wants, expectations, and constraints by discussing and negotiating boundaries. Consent necessitates active dialogue in which all parties express their desires and agree on a course of action. This communication fosters trust, and mutual understanding, and develops the emotional bond between persons.

Boundaries and Consent in Personal Growth and Self-Discovery: Encourage people to gain a thorough grasp of themselves and their desires. Individuals get an insight into their personal preferences, values, and comfort zones through defining and communicating boundaries. Consent allows people to explore their wishes and boundaries while respecting the bounds of others. This self-discovery and self-expression process fosters personal development, self-confidence, and a good sense of identity.

Setting and sustaining Healthy Relationship Dynamics: Setting and sustaining healthy relationship dynamics need boundaries and permission. They foster an atmosphere of mutual respect, equality, and justice. Power imbalances are eliminated and relationships become more balanced and equitable when people actively listen to each other's boundaries and obtain enthusiastic permission. Emotional well-being, trust, and satisfaction are all promoted by healthy relationship dynamics.

Sexual Assault and Violence Prevention: Understanding and exercising consent is a critical step in preventing sexual assault and violence. Individuals are empowered to recognize and reject non-consensual or coercive acts when the necessity of enthusiastic and continuing consent is emphasized. Promoting a culture of consent serves to challenge cultural conventions that perpetuate sexual violence and promotes a culture of respect, empathy, and understanding.

Boundaries and consent are critical for fostering healthy relationships, preventing harm, and honoring personal autonomy. They encourage open conversation, trust, and mutual understanding, while also allowing people to make educated decisions about their bodies and personal interactions. By accepting and promoting these ideals, we help to create a more secure and respected society for all.

2.2 Coping with Friendship and Peer Pressure

Friendships are a vital part of adolescence because they provide support, companionship, and possibilities for development. However, navigating friendships during this time can occasionally include dealing with peer pressure, which can impact choices and behaviors. Understanding how to negotiate friendships and deal with peer pressure is essential for sustaining good relationships and making decisions that are consistent with one's values and boundaries.

Here's a look at how to deal with friendships and peer pressure:

Recognizing Positive and Negative Influences: It is critical to understand the difference between positive and negative influences in friendships. Friends who respect limits, foster personal growth, and value individuality are positive influences. They emphasize open communication, embrace differences, and offer a secure space for people to express their thoughts and feelings. Negative influences, on the other hand, are possible.

Asserting Personal limits: It is critical to establish and communicate personal limits when navigating friendships and rejecting peer pressure. It is critical to think about one's values, views, and boundaries, and then convey them clearly to friends. Setting limits protects one's well-being and ensures mutual respect in friendships. Saying "no" to activities or behaviors that do not correspond with personal beliefs, comfort levels, or safety may constitute asserting personal boundaries.

Creating a Supportive Network: Having a supportive network of friends that respect boundaries and have similar beliefs can be quite beneficial. Surrounding oneself with friends who elevate, encourage, and understand one's choices promotes a positive and powerful environment. environment. Having a network of friends who value consent, communicate honestly, and respect personal limits provides an environment in which peer pressure is less likely to thrive.

Practicing Assertiveness and Peer Influence Resistance: It is critical to developing assertiveness skills to fight peer pressure and maintain personal boundaries. It entails expressing one's thoughts clearly, advocating personal decisions, and sticking up for oneself in difficult situations. By offering alternatives, setting firm boundaries, or seeking support from trusted friends or adults, individuals can handle peer pressure.

Developing Critical Thinking Skills: Developing critical thinking skills allows people to assess the repercussions and potential risks of peer pressure. It entails challenging assumptions, examining alternative viewpoints, and making informed judgments. Individuals can use critical thinking to understand their underlying social pressure, assess its influence on personal well-being, and make decisions that are consistent with their values and long-term aspirations.

Seeking advice and assistance from Trusted Adults: Seeking advice and assistance from trusted adults can be invaluable in difficult situations involving peer pressure. When it comes to negotiating friendships and dealing with peer pressure, parents, teachers, counselors, or mentors can provide invaluable advice, perspective, and support. These trustworthy adults may offer reassurance, assist in the exploration of alternative tactics, and enable people to make decisions that prioritize their well-being and personal beliefs.

Remember that navigating friendships and dealing with peer pressure is a process. It is common to have problems along the path, but with self-awareness, solid personal boundaries, and supportive relationships, individuals can build the resilience and skills needed to confidently navigate friendships and make decisions that align with their authentic selves

2.3   Creating   Positive   Romantic Relationships

Romantic connections are important in teenage development because they provide opportunities for connection, emotional growth, and closeness. However, it is critical to approach these partnerships with caution and understanding to promote healthy dynamics and mutual respect. The following are important factors to consider when creating healthy romantic relationships:

Self-Reflection and Understanding: It is critical to engage in self-reflection and have a firm understanding of oneself before engaging in a love relationship. This entails investigating personal beliefs, desires, and boundaries. Individuals can make intentional decisions about the type of relationship they seek and the qualities they value in a partner by recognizing their own needs and preferences.

Communication and Active Listening: Healthy love relationships are built on effective communication. It entails expressing emotions, needs, and concerns openly and politely. Active listening, on the other hand, requires hearing and comprehending one's partner's point of view. Couples can establish trust, resolve problems, and nurture emotional connection by encouraging open and honest conversation.

Mutual Respect and Equality: A healthy romantic relationship is built on mutual respect and equality. Each partner should respect and value the other's emotions, opinions, and boundaries. It is critical to respect one another's autonomy, personal space, and decision-making processes. In decision-making, power dynamics, and the distribution of responsibilities within the relationship, equality should be maintained.

Consent and Boundaries: In romantic relationships, consent, and boundaries are crucial. For any physical or intimate activity, both partners must gain unambiguous and passionate permission. It is critical to respect and honor each other's comfort levels and desires should be discussed honestly. A physical closeness that is consensual and respectful is built on continual conversation, trust, and mutual consent.

Emotional Support and Empathy: Healthy love partnerships include mutual emotional support and empathy. Partners should listen with compassion and validate each other's feelings and experiences. Empathy assists individuals in understanding and connecting with their partner's feelings, promoting emotional intimacy and strengthening their bond.

Personal Development and Independence: It is critical to retain personal development and independence when in a love relationship. Each partner should have their own set of interests, ambitions, and opportunities for self-improvement. Encouragement and support for each other's progress build a stable foundation and enables personal fulfillment inside the relationship.

Resolution of Conflicts and Compromise: Conflict is an unavoidable aspect of any relationship. Effective conflict resolution skills and a willingness to compromise are required in healthy romantic partnerships. Approaching disagreements with patience, active listening, and a problem-solving perspective is critical. Couples can work through obstacles and develop stronger together by pursuing win-win solutions and valuing the relationship over individual egos.

Shared Values and Future Planning: It is critical for long-term compatibility to align values and future ambitions. To ensure that partners are on the same page, they should share their goals, objectives, and expectations. Sharing values creates harmony, decreases conflicts, and aids in the construction of a future together.

Spotting Warning Signs and Seeking Help: It is critical in healthy romantic relationships to notice warning signals of unhealthy or abusive behavior. These may include controlling conduct, a lack of respect for boundaries, emotional manipulation, or any type of physical or emotional abuse are all indications. To protect safety and well-being, it is critical to seek help from trusted friends, family, or professionals if such warning indications appear.

Remember that healthy romantic relationships include ongoing effort, open communication, and mutual development. Individuals can build meaningful and gratifying interactions that promote their personal and emotional well-being by strengthening these foundations.

2.4 Capabilities for Effective Communication

Effective communication is the foundation of effective relationships, giving room for people to express themselves clearly, actively listen, and comprehend one another's needs and viewpoints. Building trust, settling problems, and creating emotional connections all require excellent communication skills.

Here are some essential components of good communication:

Active listening is a fundamental ability that exhibits attentiveness and empathy. It entails paying complete attention to the speaker, maintaining eye contact, and offering your undivided attention. Active listening is not just hearing what is said but also comprehending the emotions, underlying messages, and nonverbal signs. Individuals can create a secure and supportive environment for communication by demonstrating genuine interest and reflecting on what is said.

Clear and Assertive Expression: The ability to express oneself clearly and assertively is essential for good communication. It entails expressing one's thoughts, feelings, and requirements directly and courteously. Using "I" sentences might help you convey your feelings and experiences without blaming or condemning others. Being particular and avoiding generalizations ensures that messages are transmitted accurately, boosting comprehension and avoiding misconceptions.

Nonverbal cues, such as facial expressions, body language, and tone of voice, have a substantial impact on communication. Paying attention to and properly utilizing nonverbal cues improves the overall message being conveyed. Maintaining an open and relaxed posture, making adequate eye contact, and speaking in a calm and courteous tone can all help you communicate effectively nonverbally.

Empathy and Validation: Empathy is the ability to comprehend and share another person's feelings. Validating the feelings of others, these experiences contribute to the creation of a supportive environment. Empathy entails acknowledging and accepting other people's points of view, even if they differ from one's own. Validating emotions demonstrates that one appreciates and cherishes the feelings of another person, establishing trust and emotional connection.

Open-Mindedness and Respect for Differences: Effective communication requires being open-minded and accepting of different points of view. It necessitates carefully listening to many points of view, considering alternate opinions, and abstaining from judgment or defensiveness. Accepting differences and viewing them as opportunities for growth and learning improves communication and promotes open discourse.

Conflict Resolution: Conflict is an inevitable component of all relationships, and effective communication is critical to resolve disagreements constructively. Active listening, calm expression, and the use of "I" statements can all help to de-escalate heated situations. Taking it in turn to speaking up, focusing on the problem at hand rather than personal assaults, and seeking mutually beneficial solutions are all essential components of conflict resolution.

Timing and Patience: Timing is crucial in good communication. Choosing the correct time to engage in talks or address sensitive topics can lead to more fruitful discussions. Patience is also required to allow each person to completely express themselves without interruptions or haste. Allowing time and space for reflection and processing can result in more deliberate and meaningful communication.

Feedback and Validation: Giving constructive feedback and validation improves communication and supports relationship progress. Giving comments in a helpful and non-critical manner aids in the resolution of issues or places for improvement. Similarly, supporting and recognizing the viewpoints and contributions of others maintains a sense of worth, it also encourages positive conversation dynamics.

Communication is a talent that may be acquired and polished over time through continuous learning and adaptation. It necessitates continuous learning, self-reflection, and modification. Individuals can consistently develop their capacity to connect and relate to people by being open to feedback, actively researching ways to improve communication skills, and being receptive to new communication strategies.

Individuals can foster healthy and meaningful relationships, strengthen emotional attachments, and handle challenges with more understanding and empathy by learning these effective communication skills. Effective communication is the cornerstone for developing trust, settling problems, and cultivating deep and lasting relationships with others.

2.5 Recognizing and Dealing with Unhealthy Relationships or Abuse

Recognizing and dealing with dysfunctional relationships or abuse is critical for persons' well-being and safety. Understanding the warning signs of an unhealthy relationship and being aware of the many types of abuse is critical for taking the right action.

The following crucial points:

Red Flags: Being aware of red flags might assist individuals in recognizing early indicators of an unhealthy relationship. Controlling conduct, excessive jealousy, possessiveness, isolation from friends and family, disrespect, manipulation, or frequent criticism are all red flags. Individuals who pay attention to these warning indicators can examine the dynamics of the relationship and make informed judgments.

Understanding Different Types of Abuse: Abuse can appear in a variety of forms; it is critical to recognize them to protect oneself or others. Physical abuse (hitting, slapping, or pushing), emotional and verbal abuse (constant criticism, humiliation, or threats), sexual abuse (including non-consensual or forced sexual acts), financial abuse (controlling finances or restricting access to money), and digital abuse (monitoring online activities or using technology to intimidate or harass) are examples of common forms of abuse. Understanding the many types of abuse allows people to recognize when they are suffering or witnessing abusive conduct.

Trusting Your Instincts: When it comes to recognizing and dealing with toxic relationships or abuse, trusting one's instincts is critical. Listen to your inner voice if something feels off or unpleasant in your relationship. Often, individuals may downplay or might ignore warning signs, but acknowledging and honoring one's instincts is a necessary step toward prioritizing one's safety and well-being.

Seeking Help: When suffering from an unhealthy relationship or abuse, it is critical to seek help from trusted friends, family members, or experts. These people can offer valuable advice, perspectives, and emotional support. Helplines, counselors, and local groups specializing in domestic violence or relationship abuse may also be part of a support network. They can provide assistance, safety preparation, and resources to assist persons in navigating difficult situations.

Creating a Safety Plan: Individuals in abusive relationships should create a safety plan. This strategy could include locating safe locations, telling trusted others about the situation, documenting evidence of abuse, and preparing for future emergencies. A safety strategy is designed for the individual's particular circumstances and seeks to assure their physical and emotional well-being.

Setting Limits and Developing Self-Care: When coping with an unhealthy relationship or abuse, it is critical to establish limits. Clear and clear boundaries aid in the protection of personal well-being and the establishment of acceptable conduct limitations. It is also critical to prioritize self-care and seek out activities that promote emotional healing and resilience. Self-care methods like counseling, meditation, exercise, or creative outlets can help with rehabilitation.

Taking Action: It takes guts and resolves to take action to confront an unhealthy relationship or abuse. This could include getting legal assistance, engaging law enforcement if required, or seeking counseling or therapy. It is critical to realize that leaving an abusive relationship can be a complicated process, individuals should have access to the necessary resources and assistance to ensure their safety during the journey.

Remember that everyone has the right to be in a healthy and secure relationship. Recognizing the indications of an unhealthy relationship or abuse and acting to resolve them is a courageous step toward reclaiming personal well-being and creating a future free of suffering.

Chapter 3

Exploring Sexuality and Making Informed Choices

3.1 Understanding Sexual Desires, Feelings, and Fantasies.

Sexual cravings, sensations, and fantasies are all natural and unique experiences that influence a person's sexuality. Understanding and exploring these facets of one's sexuality can aid in personal development, self-discovery, and the formation of healthy sexual relationships. The purpose of this chapter is to offer insight and assistance in understanding and negotiating sexual impulses, sensations, and fantasies. Consider the following crucial points:

Accepting Sexual Diversity: Sexual wants, sensations, and fantasies include a diverse spectrum of experiences and preferences. It is critical to understand that everyone's desires and fantasies are unique and might differ drastically. There is no one "normal" or "right" way to experience or express one's sexuality. Accepting sexual variety and realizing that individual wants are unique, Valid, and can contribute to a healthy and inclusive attitude to sexuality exploration.

Self-Awareness and Reflection: Understanding one's sexual wants, feelings, and fantasies requires developing self-awareness. Reflecting on one's personal experiences, exploring one's thoughts and feelings, and detecting patterns or triggers can all provide significant insights into one's desires. Self-reflection allows people to better understand their sexual preferences, boundaries, and what gives them pleasure.

Communication and Consent: Navigating sexual desires, sensations, and fantasies requires effective communication and consent. It is critical to openly communicate wishes and boundaries with a partner to develop a consensual and respectful sexual connection. Consent should always be freely, joyfully, and explicitly granted, and it should last the whole of any sexual interaction. Respecting and honoring a partner's limits and wants is also part of consent.

Understanding the Difference Between Fantasy and Reality: It is critical to understand the difference between sexual fantasies and real-life wants. Fantasies are imagined scenarios or thoughts that may or may not mirror the actual goals or intentions of the individual. It is critical to understand that imagination does not always transfer into real-life actions or preferences. Exploring and accepting dreams can be a healthy component of one's sexual expression if they are consistent with the ideals of consent and respect for oneself and others.

Managing Guilt or Shame: Sexual desires, thoughts, and fantasies can occasionally elicit feelings of guilt or shame. Remember that consensual and ethical sexual expression is a normal and healthy component of adulthood. Recognizing and dealing with any guilt or shame related to sexual cravings can entail self-compassion, seeking support from trusted individuals or professionals, and knowing that healthy sexual expression is a personal and subjective experience.

Personal Limits and Limits: Understanding and setting personal limits is critical in navigating sexual desires, sensations, and fantasies. Boundaries assist individuals in defining their comfort zones, communicating their limitations to partners, and ensuring that sexual encounters are consistent with their values and preferences. Setting and maintaining boundaries helps individuals to prioritize their well-being and engage in consensual and mutually enjoyable sexual activities.

Exploration and Consent in Relationships: In a consenting and trustworthy relationship, exploring sexual wants, sensations, and fantasies can be an enriching feature. Partners can have open and honest discussions about their desires and fantasies, making sure that both partners are at ease and excited about the adventure. The establishment of trust and consent fosters a safe and happy sexual environment.

Seeking Professional Help: If people have problems or questions about their sexual wants, feelings, or fantasies, they can seek help from specialists such as therapists, counselors, or sexual health experts. These specialists can offer a nonjudgmental and encouraging environment in which to express issues, obtain insights, and resolve any challenges or fears.

Remember that each person's sexual urges, feelings, and dreams are unique and personal. Consent, communication, and respect for yourself and your partners should always be prioritized when understanding and exploring these elements of your sexuality. Maintaining a healthy and successful sexual life necessitates continual self-reflection, open-mindedness, and dedication.

3.2   Masturbation: Recognizing   and Accepting Self-Pleasure

Masturbation is a normal and widespread feature of human sexuality. It entails self-stimulating to have sexual pleasure. Understanding and accepting masturbation has various advantages, including self-discovery, stress alleviation, and the development of a healthy relationship with one's own body. In this section, we shall go deeper into the subject of masturbation. Consider the following crucial points:

Masturbation Must Be Normalized: First and foremost, masturbation must be seen as a healthy and natural element of human sexuality. Masturbation is a personal choice that varies from person to person. It is critical to understand that masturbation does not reflect negatively on a person's character, values, or relationships. It is a personal and personal activity that can provide enjoyment and contentment.

Self-Exploration and Body Awareness: Masturbation allows people to explore their bodies, learn about their erogenous zones, and discover what they find pleasurable. It raises body awareness and helps people understand their distinct sexual responses. Individuals can become more attuned to their desires, preferences, and boundaries by indulging in self-pleasure, which can improve their sexual experiences both alone and with others.

Sexual Health and Well-Being: Masturbation provides a variety of physical and mental benefits. It can be used to naturally reduce sexual tension and stress. It can also help with better sleep, a better mood, and less anxiety. Masturbation can be an effective self-care and self-soothing tool, enhancing overall sexual health and well-being.

Communication and learning: Masturbation can give people crucial information about their own bodies and sexual responses. Individuals can obtain knowledge about what they enjoy and communicate their wishes more successfully with partners by discovering their pleasure through masturbation. Understanding and expressing one's sexual preferences can result in more fulfilling sexual encounters in both solo and partnered situations.

Personal Safety and Safer Sex: Masturbation is a low-risk sexual behavior. It carries no danger of sexually transmitted infections (STIs) or unwanted pregnancy. Individuals who wish to abstain from sexual activity with partners or who are not yet ready for sexual intimacy may benefit from solo sexual exploration. It gives a private and safe space for sexual expression.

Overcoming Shame and Guilt: Because of cultural, religious, or personal views, some people may feel shame or guilt about masturbation. Masturbation is a natural and healthy element of human sexuality, and it is vital to challenge and conquer these unpleasant emotions. Recognizing that self-indulgence can be a pleasant and rewarding practice might assist folks in letting go of any unneeded guilt or shame.

Privacy and Personal Comfort: It is critical to provide a safe and comfortable setting for masturbation. Individuals must find a secluded location where they can relax and feel at ease to truly appreciate the event. Individuals can embrace their self-pleasure without constraint or distraction by ensuring privacy and taking steps to feel secure and comfortable.

Remember that masturbating is a personal choice Individual comfort levels and preferences may differ. Self-pleasure must be done with consent, respect for personal limits, and an emphasis on self-care. Accepting masturbation as a normal and healthy part of your sexuality will help you have a more fulfilled and satisfied sexual life.

3.3 Contraception and Safe Sex Practices

Engaging in safe sex practices and using effective contraception techniques are critical for minimizing the risk of unwanted pregnancies and sexually transmitted infections (STIs). This section will provide information on various safe sex practices and contraception techniques to assist individuals in making educated sexual health decisions. Consider the following crucial points:

Condoms: Condoms are a popular and effective means of contraception. They act as a barrier to the interchange of bodily fluids, lowering the risk of both pregnancy and STIs. During vaginal, anal, and oral sex, condoms should be used regularly and appropriately. Choose high-quality condoms, verify the expiration date, and keep them in a cold, dry area.

Hormonal Contraception: Hormonal methods of contraception, such as birth control pills, patches, injections, and hormonal intrauterine devices (IUDs), prevent conception by regulating hormones. When utilized appropriately and regularly, these strategies are quite effective. They do not, however, protect against STIs. It is critical to talk with a healthcare practitioner to choose the best hormonal strategy for you depending on your specific health needs and lifestyle.

Other barrier methods, such as diaphragms, cervical caps, and contraceptive sponges, provide a physical barrier to prevent sperm from reaching the cervix in addition to condoms. These treatments can be combined with spermicide to boost their efficiency. For proper insertion, removal, and maintenance of various barrier technologies, it is critical to follow the guidelines provided by healthcare professionals.

Long-Acting Reversible Contraception (LARCs): Long-acting reversible contraception, such as hormonal and non-hormonal IUDs and contraceptive implants, provide very effective and convenient contraception choices. Once implanted, they provide continuous pregnancy protection for a duration ranging from several months to several years. LARCs require professional insertion and removal and are appropriate for anyone looking for long-term contraception.

Emergency contraception, also known as the "morning-after pill," is a backup strategy used to prevent pregnancy following unprotected intercourse or contraceptive failure. It is most effective when taken as soon as possible after intercourse, but it can be used within a certain interval following intercourse. Many nations have over-the-counter emergency contraception, which should be used sparingly as a backup technique rather than as a regular type of contraception.

STI Prevention: It is critical to practice safe sex by utilizing barrier techniques, such as condoms, during sexual activity to lower the risk of STIs. Regular STI testing is critical for early discovery and treatment, especially for people who have several partners or are in new sexual relationships. To maintain a secure and healthy sexual environment, open and honest discussion about sexual health with partners is vital.

Dual Protection: Using both contraception and barrier techniques (e.g., condoms) at the same time provides dual protection against pregnancy and STIs. This method is indicated for people who are not in a mutually monogamous relationship or who are unsure about their partner's sexual health history. Dual protection provides a holistic approach to sexual health while reducing hazards.

Consultation with Healthcare Professionals: When making a decision, it is best to speak with a healthcare professional, such as a gynecologist or a family planning clinic, who can provide individualized advice based on specific health considerations and preferences. They can assist in determining the best procedures, discussing any adverse effects, and ensuring correct usage and maintenance.

Remember that practicing safe sex and using proper contraception options are critical for maintaining your sexual health and well-being. Individuals who are aware and proactive can make responsible decisions that are in line with their particular preferences and lifestyle while limiting the possibility of unforeseen effects.

3.4 Preventing Sexually Transmitted Infections (STIs)

Sexually transmitted infections (STIs) are illnesses that can be passed from person to person through sexual contact. They pose severe health hazards and, if untreated, can have long-term effects. Understanding sexually transmitted infections (STIs), their modes of transmission, and preventative techniques is critical for sustaining sexual health. This section will include information on common STIs as well as preventative techniques.

Sexually Transmitted Diseases (STIs)

a) *Human Immunodeficiency Virus (HIV):* HIV damages the immune system, rendering people more vulnerable to infections and illnesses. It is primarily transferred by unprotected sexual contact, sharing needles, or transmission from mother to child during childbirth or breastfeeding.

b) *Chlamydia* is a bacterial infection that can harm the reproductive organs. It can be passed on via vaginal, anal, or oral intercourse.

c) *Gonorrhea:* Gonorrhea is a bacterial infection that, if left untreated, can lead to consequences. It is primarily spread through unprotected sexual contact.

d) *Syphilis:* Syphilis is a bacterial infection that develops in stages and can damage a variety of body systems. It is spread through direct contact with syphilis sores, which usually occur during sexual intercourse.

e) *Genital Herpes:* Genital herpes is a viral illness that causes sores or blisters on the genitals or nearby locations. During sexual activity, it is spread through skin-to-skin contact.

f) *Human Papillomavirus (HPV):* HPV is a virus that causes genital warts and several types of cancer. It is spread through sexual contact, which includes vaginal, anal, and oral intercourse.

g) *Hepatitis B and C:* These are viral illnesses that mostly impact the liver. They can be passed from mother to kid after childbirth or during unprotected sexual intercourse.

STIs can be transferred through a variety of sexual behaviors, including vaginal, anal, and oral intercourse. Some STIs can also be spread nonsexual, such as through the sharing of contaminated needles or mother-to-child transmission during childbirth or breastfeeding.

Prevention Strategies:

a) Abstinence: The most effective strategy to avoid STIs is to refrain from sexual activity.

b) Condom Use: Using condoms correctly and consistently during sexual intercourse can dramatically lower the risk of STI transmission.

c) Vaccination: Vaccines for specific STIs, such as HPV and hepatitis B, are available. These infections can be avoided with vaccination.

c) STI Testing: STI testing should be done regularly especially crucial for those who have several sexual partners or are in new sexual relationships. STI testing enables early detection and therapy.

e) discussion and Trust: Maintaining a safe sexual environment requires open and honest discussion with sexual partners about STI history, testing, and preventative strategies.

f) Reducing the Number of Sexual Partners Reducing the number of sexual partners and practicing mutual monogamy with a partner who has tested negative for STIs can lower the risk of exposure.

g) Safe Injection Practices When injecting drugs, use sterile needles and avoid sharing injection equipment to avoid the spread of blood-borne illnesses such as HIV and hepatitis.

h) Prenatal Care: Pregnant women should receive regular prenatal care to screen for and prevent STI transmission from mother to child.

The Value of Early Diagnosis and Treatment

Early detection and treatment of STIs are critical for reducing problems and future transmission. Individuals who fear they may have an STI or have been exposed to one should seek medical assistance and get tested as soon as possible.

Remember that safe sex, the use of barrier techniques such as condoms, and open conversation with sexual partners are critical to decreasing the risk of STIs. Maintaining sexual health requires regular STI testing and obtaining medical care when necessary.

3.5 Making Informed Sexual Activity and Readiness Decisions

Making informed sexual activity decisions and establishing one's preparedness are critical parts of healthy sexual development. It entails comprehending personal beliefs, desires, and boundaries, as well as taking into account elements such as emotional readiness, permission, and communication. This section will help you make informed judgments about sexual activity and measure your readiness.

The following are crucial points:

Self-Reflection: Use self-reflection to gain a better understanding of your values, beliefs, and attitudes around sex. Consider your mental and physical preparedness, personal boundaries, and the reasons behind your desires. It is critical, to be honest with oneself and to investigate your comfort zones and boundaries.

Emotional Preparedness: Evaluate your emotional preparedness for sexual activity. Sexual closeness can be a very personal and intimate experience. Make sure you're prepared to deal with the emotional complications that may develop from sexual engagement, such as feelings of attachment, vulnerability, and closeness.

Communication and Consent: In any sexual relationship, open and honest communication is essential. It is critical to be able to express your desires, boundaries, and concerns to your spouse. Consent must always be gained and honored. Keep in mind that consent is a continuous process that can be given or withdrawn at any time during sexual activity.

Education and Awareness: Learn about sexual health, contraception techniques, and the risks of sexual activity. Keep up to date on sexually transmitted diseases (STIs), pregnancy prevention, and the value of frequent check-ups. Knowledge allows you to make informed judgments and take action.

Recognize and resist peer pressure and societal expectations around sexual activity Do not engage in sexual activities just to please others or to fit in. Your decisions should reflect your ideals, degree of comfort, and personal well-being.

Consider the characteristics of your relationship, as well as the level of trust and communication with your partner. Mutual respect, trust, and a common awareness of boundaries and expectations are required for a healthy sexual relationship. Before engaging in sexual activity, make sure you have a firm foundation of trust and open communication.

Personal Boundaries: Identify and define your sexual activity boundaries. Boundaries can include the types of sexual activities you are comfortable with, the speed with which you wish to advance, and the level of closeness you are comfortable with. Communicate your boundaries to your spouse explicitly, and respect theirs as well.

Seeking Advice: If you have any questions or concerns, seek advice from trusted adults, healthcare professionals, or reputable information sources. They can offer assistance, answer your questions, and assist you in making informed decisions that are best for you.

Remember that sexual engagement is a personal decision that should be based on educated choices, consent, and personal preparation. Take the time to get to know yourself, speak openly, and put your physical and mental well-being first. Your sexual experience is unique, and you must navigate it in a way that feels natural to you.

Conclusion

Congratulations! You have completed this book on sex education for girls. We have covered a wide range of issues in these chapters, from understanding puberty and its bodily changes to building healthy relationships, exploring sexual impulses, and making educated decisions regarding sexual behavior. We've covered vital facts to provide you with knowledge and assist you navigate your sexual development path with confidence and understanding.

Remember that understanding your body, emotions, and boundaries is essential for developing a healthy and meaningful sex life. Puberty brings about substantial physical and emotional changes, and it is crucial to accept and enjoy these changes as a normal part of growing up.

We've talked about how important consent, boundaries, and good communication are in building respectful relationships. Recognizing and dealing with toxic relationships or abuse is critical for your health and safety.

We've also covered themes like sexual cravings, dreams, and the impact of hormones, all to encourage you to explore and understand your sexuality without judgment. Accepting self-satisfaction, engaging in safe sex, and understanding contraception techniques are all important components of preserving your sexual health.

Furthermore, we have shed light on sexually transmitted infections (STIs), their prevention, and the importance of STI testing regularly. You can protect yourself and your relationships by understanding the hazards and taking the required safeguards.

The most crucial component of your sexual adventure is ultimately your agency. You have the right to make educated decisions about your body, preferences, and sexual readiness. Believe in yourself and pay attention. Remember that the basis of healthy sexual relationships is consent, communication, and mutual respect.

Don't be afraid to seek advice from trusted adults, healthcare professionals, or support networks as you continue on your road of self-discovery and sexual development. It is good to ask questions, seek answers, and embrace the growth that comes with your sexual well-being as a lifelong adventure.

Above all, be kind to yourself and others. Accept diversity, value differences, and foster a culture of consent and inclusivity. You are helping to create a world where everyone can have healthy, satisfying, and respectful relationships.

May this book be a beneficial resource for you as you negotiate the complexity of sex education with confidence, awareness, and a strong feeling of self-worth, embrace your sexuality. Remember that you have power over your own body and decisions and that you deserve to be loved, respected, and happy in all aspects of your life.

I wish you a fulfilling and empowered journey of sexual exploration and personal development!

With best wishes,

[Morgane Lee Rice]